HOW TO CURE DIABETES

A GUIDE TO CURE DIABETES WITH NATURE HERBS

Copyright@2023

Giovanni Scott

TABLE OF CONTENT

CHAPTER ONE

DIABETES MELLITUS: A CHECK ON NATURE

Diabetes is a chronic disease that occurs either when the pancreas does not produce enough insulin or when the body cannot effectively use the insulin it produces. People are diabetic till death and only go from bad to worse due to the side effects of some drugs. Sure you will be seeing improvements as you are taking the drugs but whether you like it or not, the side effects are there. The drugs are known to cause kidney damage, liver damage, heart damage etc. Once you start medication for diabetes, it

becomes a journey that never ends
and only get worse. It starts with
feeling sluggish and being overweight
but why, simply because you are
trapped in a cycle.

When you eat your body makes
insulin, cell resist insulin, sugar will
be stored as fat, so you will keep
gaining weight and getting tired
always. Though, not all diabetes
patients are also thin. Some are
overweight and still suffer from the
disease. Initial perception is that only
obese individuals are susceptible to
diabetes. This is contrary to reality.
Even thin individuals are affected by
it. Those who are thin due to diabetes
are those who were aware of their

condition in a timely manner. When irresponsible individuals become emaciated, the disease may have affected their vital organs, such as liver and kidney. Therefore, it is advised that we take tests frequently. There are local remedies that can cure it before the liver and kidneys are affected. In addition, diabetics can consume certain carbohydrates without negative adverse effects. Examples include oat meal, immature plantain, cocoyam with a brownish hue, jute, okra, and other vegetables. Patients with diabetes must not overeat. They must not consume an excessive amount of water in the evening. They must consume supper by 7 p.m. Patients with diabetes are permitted to ingest five or more foods each day, but every meal has to be tiny. Essential are detoxification and weight management. Because sugar/glucose is not the underlying cause, the majority of diabetics who rely on medication do not improve. The underlying cause is diabetes mellitus. Gaining weight is a sign of insulin resistance. Glucose is an essential nutrient that improves and energizes blood cells. It is incorporated into the organism and transported to various cells via the blood. The excess is retained in the brain for later use or excreted through the bladder if the concentration becomes toxic. Insulin is the hormone responsible for transporting glucose to cells. It is manufactured by the pancreas. Insulin is important for modulating the level of glucose in the blood. Diabetes is a metabolic disease characterized by elevated glucose levels (sugar). Normal blood glucose levels are less than 140 milligrams per deciliter.

TYPES OF DIABETES

1. TYPE 1: Occurs when the pancreas produces little or no glucose. it is also known as metabolism diabetes because it occurs when the immune system stacks the cells in the pancreas that produce insulin thereby allowing blood sugar level to rise. This type of diabetes occurs mostly from childhood or early adulthood.

2. TYPE 2: is a condition in which the body cells refuse or unable to use the insulin produced by the pancreas, then it over work the pancreas by producing more insulin and may eventually breakdown. Occasionally known as non-mellitus. This kind of diabetes is largely caused by excessive body fat and lifestyle. Type 1 is the defect of the pancreas while type 2 is the defect of the cells.

3. Gestational diabetes: is the increase in blood glucose of a pregnant woman. This form of diabetes is caused by hormones that inhibit insulin production all through infertility. people should monitor this during pregnancy as it can lead to complications for the mother and the baby. It usually goes away after delivery but the mother and the child are at risk of having type 2 diabetes in the future.

CAUSES OF DIABETES

- Obesity
- Poor diet
- Family history
- Old age
- Nutritional deficiency
- Sugary foods and others

SYMPTOMS OF DIABETES

- Belly fat
- Blurry vision
- Frequent urination
- Frequent desire to drink water
- Numbness in the upper and lower limb
- Fatigue
- High blood sugar
- Wound takes longer to heal

HOW TO MANAGE DIABETES

- Do more exercise.
- Consume healthy food always
- Eat more vegetables and fruits

- Take a lemon with a tablespoon of honey in a glass cup of water early in the morning daily

- Drink fennel tea daily

- Taking herbs like Bitter melon, turmeric, India gooseberry, holy basil, fenugreek, bill berry, humbelletta, insulin plant, cinnamon etc.

Things to avoid

- White rice

- Bread

- Beverages

- Pasta

- Reduce crab intake

- Sugary foods

- Flavors and the likes

CHAPTER TWO

FOOD DIET FOR DIABETES PATIENT

When having to deal with managing blood sugar levels, obsessing over everything you cannot have may seem your best option. But while it is certainly improvement to limit foods white, refined breeds, pasta and fried fatty foods, paying attention to what you should eat is just as vital.

The ingredients below havc been singled out by numerous nutritionists and diabetes experts. What makes these foods exceptionally great is that they are packed with four healthy nutrients: fiber, omega – 3, calcium and vitamin D, all of which are essential to a diabetic. They are also incredibly versatile. You can add them to your meals, eat them as stand-alone snacks, or add them to recipes.

1. BEANS:

Besides being high in fibers, beans contain plant compounds that help you feel full, provide steady blood sugar and are low in cholesterols. And while not packed in calcium, you will get a good enough dose. Have a cup of white beans will get you almost 100mg of calcium, making up about 10%of your daily intakes.

USE: Beans can be added to salads, soups, chili and more. There's a variety of beans available, so you are not restricted to eating the same type twice.

2. DIARY:

Diabetics can include milk, cottage cheese, and yogurt in their nutrition as a rich source of vitamin D and calcium. In fact, one study found that woman who consumed more than 1,200mg of calcium and more than 800UI (international unit) of vitamin D a day were 33% less by to advance diabetes than those not taking enough.

USE: Select yogurt or cottage cheese as a snack or dessert, and use milk to make oatmeal or to thicken soups.

3. BARLEY: Barley is rich in a special kind of soluble fiber called beta – glycan, which according to research can lower total and LDL cholesterol by preventing your body's ability to absorb it. One review found that consuming just 3 grams a day (a single serving of barley) can lower cholesterol by 8%. As a result of its high fiber content, barley can also help steady your blood sugar. The grain also contains a modest amount of calcium.

USE:

Select hulled barley which is not as refined as pearl barley. Soak it immediate, then add to soups, stews or rice pilaf.

4. OATS

Aside from containing an essential source of fiber content (a half cup

provides 4g) oats help lower LDL
cholesterol and improve insulin
resistance. The soluble fiber in oats
slow the rate at which your body can
breakdown and absorb carbohydrates,
enabling your blood sugar levels to
stay stable.

USE

Eat oats every morning as part of your
breakfast. You can also take it as
snack wirh all kinds of recipes from
pancakes to meatloaf and cookies too.

5. BERRIES

Berries are loaded with fiber (a cup of
black berries contain 7.6g of fiber)
and antioxidants called polyphenols.
A 2008 study published in the
American Journal of clinical nutrition

found that people with heart disease risk factors, who ate berries for 8 weeks had a drop in blood pressure and a boost in good HDL cholesterol.

USE:

Mix berries into oatmeal, ice cream or salads.

6. DATES

Besides their sweet taste and delightful texture, dates supply a generous amount of fiber (7 dates contain 4g) making them a perfect diabetes friendly snacks. Dates are also packed with antioxidants, a serving of dates contain more antioxidant than oranges, grapes, broccoli and peppers.

USE

Schiff with pecan or walnut halves for a satisfying snack. You can also add them to break and cookies.

8. GREENS

When it comes to upping your intake of "greens" you are solely limited to lettuce. In fact, your choices are pretty diverse. Greens range from chips to mustard, beet greens, as well as chard. All are an outstanding source of fiber (one cooked cup contains anywhere from 3 to 10g) and calcium (supplying around 100 to 250 per cup). Aside from being beneficial to your blood sugar levels, greens are also good for your heart.

USE

Prepared well, greens can be pretty delicious. You can use them in entrees, sandwiches and salads.

9. FLAX SEED

Though they may be tiny flaxseed packs a big health punch. They are best known for their source of fiber and alpha-linoleic acid (ALA), which your body converts to omega3 in several large studies, researchers have found a link between increase ALA and lower odds of heart other cardiovascular issues. These seeds are also known to lower cholesterol and blood sugar.

USE:

Grounded flax seed may be added to all kinds of foods such as oat meal, low fat cottage cheese, and fruit smoothies.

10. WALNUTS

One ounce of these healthy nuts provides 2g of fiber and 2.6g of ALA. If you are watching your weight through, control your portion.

Peanuts butter

Studies have shown a link between peanut butter and a reduced risk of diabetes. The fiber content (2 tables spoons has almost 2g) may be a contribution factor. This classic comfort food contains mostly

monounsaturated fat, making it a
heart healthy option.

NATURAL THERAPY FOR DIABETES

We understand that as a diabetic, your diet is of utmost importance. And that sometimes those sweet craving is just way too hard to resist. So we bring you a list of natural goodies that tantalize your task buds are easy to find and as a bonus, are great for your health.

1. PEARS

Rich in potassium and loaded with fiber. A pear is also low in carbohydrates. Add them in your fruit bowl or mix it up with spinach to get an instant fix for your hunger pangs.

Despite the fact that fruits and vegetables are good for you, there's no denying the fact that some of them contain sugar and carbohydrates in small amount. So keep your portion small and do check with your nutritionist before any major diet changes.

2. CABBAGES

Cabbages has a low glycaemic index of 10 which is very diabetes friendly, it is also a rich source of vitamin C and K. However, keep an eye on the fat content. If you are including cabbage in your diet.

3. BERRIES

Tempting red strawberries or indigo colored blue berries or just any berries for that matter. Expert advice that these little colorful fruit are rich in antioxidants, vitamins and fiber and are low card. So top off your breakfast with some strawberries or just toss them in your mouth. It adds a pop of color and a dollop of health

4. ORANGES

Despite the fact that an orange contains sugar, it also contains other compounds that help control blood glucose, which makes it good for diabetes patients. The soluble fiber present in an orange thickness as it's being digested. This in turn slows down the sugar absorption, offering better control of your blood sugar.

5. BEANS

Studies have demonstrated that lentils, black beans, or kidney beans are quite beneficial for a diabetic's health. They are protein-rich and without much fat and energy. They make you feel full, slow down your digestion process and prevents blood sugar from spiking.

6. SPINACH

Research have revealed that spinach, a pure, leafy greens vegetable, contains incredibly few calories and carbohydrates. This is excellent news for diabetics. In actuality, spinach is one of the few foods a diabetic may eat nearly without restriction.

7. APPLES

Apples has few energy and carbohydrates. This transportable fruit is the ideal snack because it is simple to carry around in your backpack. This diabetes-friendly fruit, which is brimming with vitamins and antioxidants, will give your meal an extra crunch and healthful boost. Recent studies have shown that eating one apple per day can provide the body with a healthy amount of antioxidants while reducing the blood levels of dangerous cholesterol by 40%.

8. OKRA (LADY'S FINGERS)

Kids and diabetics will love this vegetable. Okra, like brinjals and oranges, is one of the finest foods to eat if you have diabetes since it contains soluble fiber.

9. BRINJAL

Non-starchy, low carbohydrate and soluble fiber, could a vegetable be more perfect for diabetes? Load up on this easily available.

10. VINEGAR

Vinegar is an excellent dietary compound responsible for diluting concentrated sugar levels in the blood studies have shown that two spoonful of vinegar before a meal can reduce the glucose influx.

11. SOY

Soy proteins are one of the miracle cures for reducing diabetes among crucial patients. There is flavored contained in them reduce the sugar content in blood and keep the body nourished while accumulating much fewer calories, when compared to other foods.

12. CINNAMON POWDER

Powdered cinnamon, apart from spicing up your foods, has the ability to lower blood sugar levels, as well take a pinch of cinnamon with warm water every day and kill diabetes goodbye.

13. USING METHI SEEDS

Fenugreek or methi seeds are considered the most effective of natural cures that can help alleviate typical symptoms of diabetes. Methi seeds must be steeped longer in water. The water concentrated with the seeds juices should be consumed early in the morning on an empty stomach. For making this natural concoction stronger, crush the seeds and sieve them through a cloth or filter paper.

14. FRESH FRUITS

Natural fruits sugars are the best options, as dietary supplements, since they provide all the necessary vitamins and minerals required. Studies have shown that an adequate intake of vitamin A and C maintain blood and bone wealth. Include fresh citrus and fruits, like oranges, apples, pineapple, grapes and lemons in your diet. Consume bananas in moderation, since their sugar structure is more complex than that of citrus fruit.

15. ASPARAGUS: Just 20 calories and a good amount of dietary fiber per saving, asparagus makes a wonderful food choice for those with diabetes. Asparagus contains an abundance of antioxidants, and its consumption is believed to reduce the risk of diabetes, heart disease, and cancer, as well as delay the ageing process.

16. BROCCOLI:

Broccoli is another excellent dinner food for diabetics to incorporate into their diet. Beta-carotene, which is abundant in phytonutrients, is known to promote healthy vision, powerful molars and bone fragments, and skin health. Additionally, it is considered that broccoli can prevent cell damage caused by elevated blood sugar.

17. CARROTS

Carrots are rich in fiber and vital micronutrients that strengthen the immune system. Carrot consumption is also believed to prevent the development of certain malignancies. In terms of diabetes, raw carrots may also reduce the risk of developing type 2 diabetes, even in those with a genetic susceptibility to the disease.

18. FRESH VEGETABLES:

Fresh vegetables are abundant in iron, zinc, potassium, calcium, and other vital nutrients. These nutrients and acids improve general circulatory and central nervous health. This causes the body to optimally absorb proteins and generate insulin.

19. JACK FRUIT: Fresh jack supper is a 3600-year-old tradition in Kerala, where it is known as chakkapuzhukku. Until the Portuguese introduced cassava plant from Brazil, it was the primary source of carbohydrates during the summer. Over the past few hundred years, the majority of Malayali have developed diabetes, which makes this inherently glutinous, prickly, but flavorful tropical food undesirable. Kerala has become the diabetes capital of Melia as a result of its use of the identical jackfruit meal recipe with cassava's starchy root in the past few centuries. In return, the Portuguese popularized the appellation chukka to jaca, and it is now widely referred to as jackfruit. A study conducted in Sri Lanka, in which Raw jack fruit is utilized as a carbohydrate substitute, revealed a significant reduction in blood sugar level three months after dinner consumption. Nonetheless, a study found that when raw jackfruit dinner is consumed for dinner by diabetic patients, their blood sugar levels and, in some instances, insulin levels decrease significantly overnight. Diabetes has reached epidemic proportions in India, and the abundant plantain may hold the key to its treatment.

20. TOMATOES FOR HYPERGLYCEMIA

The tomatoes are the fruit of the plant lycopersicon esculentum. It can also be classified as a berry as it forms a single ovary. Regulating glucose levels is an essential component of diabetes control. For diabetes, healthy glucose level can be achieved by a proper whole food diet in conjunction with stress management and exercise. Because of their low carbohydrate content, tomatoes can play a big role in controlling blood sugar level. The minimal nutritive value also can assist diabetics reduce weight by reducing their caloric intake. Tomatoes are an outstanding antioxidant source and help maintain the oxidative equilibrium of the body. Consuming foods rich in antioxidants may minimize the likelihood of diabetes-related issues in adults. Tomatoes are an abundant source of the antioxidants vitamin E and beta carotene. In addition, they have substantial amounts of phytonutrients such as flavones and carotenoids such as lycopene and lutein. These antioxidants safeguard the body by inhibiting the peroxidation of lipids. This is the oxidative degradation of lipids in the bloodstream or cell membranes. Antioxidants also safeguard the body by enhancing the activity of enzymes. Diabetes-afflicted kidneys are protected by the antioxidant properties of tomatoes, according to studies. Numerous patients also suffer from cardiovascular conditions. Tomatoes contain numerous nutrients that support the vascular system. There are two primary research avenues that link tomatoes to a healthy body. The first entails antioxidant support, whereas the second explores blood fat regulation. The heart is accountable for circulating blood, which carries oxygen throughout the body. Antioxidants play an essential part in preventing oxygen-induced damage.

Here, tomatoes contain high concentrations of vitamins C and E. Tomatoes perform a crucial role in preventing oxidative damage. Lycopene is another nutrient present in tomatoes that is beneficial to the heart. Lycopene can reduce the level of lipid peroxidation in the blood. Lipid peroxidation is the process by which lipids in the blood or cell membranes become oxidized and damaged. The body's immune system responds to these injuries by initiating a chain of reactions that can eventually obstruct the arteries. Lycopene prevents this damage from taking place. The second line of inquiry investigates the relationship between tomatoes and the regulation of blood lipids. Tomato-rich diets have been shown to enhance the blood fat profile. Triglyceride and total cholesterol levels both decrease. In macrophage cells, lycopene inhibits the accumulation of cholesterol molecules. These cells are forms of white blood cells, and the triglycerides they gather contributes to the development of atherosclerosis. Blood cells known as platelets are another way in which tomatoes promote cardiac health. Platelets aid in blood coagulation, and excessive platelet levels can lead to blood clots and blockages. Platelets tend to adhere excessively in diabetics, resulting in excessive coagulation. This is why people with diabetes are susceptible to stroke and cardiac disease. Tomatoes contain numerous phytonutrients that reduce the tendency of platelets to clump together, thereby lowering the risk of blood vessel blockage. Combined with the other benefits to the heart described above, tomatoes' ability to regulate platelet aggregation makes them a highly effective means of maintaining heart health. Both systolic and diastolic blood pressure can decrease in diabetics who consume approximately 200 grams of fresh tomatoes, according to research. Other nutrients produced by tomatoes can alter the metabolic activity of prostate cancer cells. It can also induce programmed cell death (aproptosis) in fully formed prostate cancer cells. Identical outcomes have been observed in cases of non-small cell lung carcinoma. Studies have demonstrated that lycopene can reduce the risk of developing breast cancer. Studies have demonstrated that diets rich in tomatoes reduce the risk of developing neurological diseases such as Alzheimer's. Numerous studies have found a correlation between tomato-rich diets and a lower risk of obesity. Other essential nutrients in tomatoes include:

- **Vitamin K:** It helps promote good bone health Vitamin B1, B2 & B6 – help promote heart

- **Molybdenum:** Promotes enzyme production

- **Chromium and manganese:** Helps balance blood sugar

- **Iron:** Healthy blood

- **Phosphorus and copper:** Promotes good bone health.

- **Proteins;** Helps build muscles with all these numerous benefits, it is no surprise that tomatoes are recommended by dietitians for diabetic patients.

Using Natural Juices

Some juices have been found to be effective in controlling high sugar levels that can prove fatal for diabetes. These are juices of fruits and vegetables that are further enriched with anti-oxidants and many rare micro nutrients. The most recommended variety here is the Bitter Gourd or Karela juice. Other options include grape juice or the juice like extract made from boiling mango leaves in water.

1. Aloe-Gel: An effective natural concoction for diabetes can be prepared by adding a few teaspoons of grounded Bay leaf with one teaspoon of turmeric. This mixture should be mixed with an equal amount of Aloe-Vera gel and consumed daily before lunch and dinner.

2. Chapattis: Another useful way of managing diabetes is increasing the daily intake of fiber in the natural form. This includes increasing the fiber content in chapattis that tend to be eaten with regularity in Indian homes. The refined flour should be mixed with a combination of flours procured from different cereals, particularly those high in soluble fiber. This includes flours of barley and lentils like cheng Dal and soya bean.

3. Jarul or Banaba: Diabetics can use Banaba or jarul plant extract. Banana is among the lesser known of herbal plant in Indian. Along with Indian it is grown in only a handful of other nations. The herbal powder of Banaba extract can be used to make herbal tea. This plants contains high concentration of corosolic acid the most potent of biochemical compounds that stimulate faster glucose metabolism and help to regulate blood sugar and insulin levels that is very useful for combating diabetes.

4. Jamun: jamun is one of the rarest plants where nearly each part, the leaves, berry and seeds are known to help in controlling blood sugar levels.

5. Neem leaves: are also useful in a similar manner instead of using only neem leaves, you can also add leaves of Tusil and Bel Patra. These leaves can be steamed together just to increase the efficacy of the extracted liquid. Amla, also known as the Indian gooseberry, is similarly effective at regulating glucose levels.

6. Pawpaw foliage juice:

Pawpaw leaf fluid controls hormone secretion, which in turn controls blood sugar. It contains potent antioxidants that reduce diabetes-related complications such as kidney injury and fatty liver. This beverage can effectively treat diabetes.

Preparation

Extract the fluid from sufficient pawpaw leaves.

CHAPTER THREE

Diabetes has become one of the most widespread new pandemics and one of the quickest diseases in the globe. This is largely due to the unhealthy diet and practices fostered by current living. Everyone should be aware of the symptoms of type 2 diabetes since the most effective method to prevent the disease is to detect it early and take defensive measures. Pre-diabetes is the general term for these conditions. The blood sugar levels are not yet at the stage of full-blown diabetes, and the condition is still curable. Initially, familiarize yourself with the following symptoms:

- Feeling parched despite consuming copious amounts of fluids

- Feeling sluggish despite adequate hours of rest

- Peeing more regularly, particularly at night

- Putting on weight notwithstanding no dietary changes or physical exercise

- Getting famished minutes after consuming;

- Skin conditions that require a great deal of time to recover;

- Distorted night vision

- Getting extremely fatigued

When recognize pair or more of those signs, it is imperative that you undergo testing to determine if you are on the road to developing diabetes. Essentially, there are two exams available:

1. Fast plasma glucose test:

Fasting for 8 to 10 hours earlier to the fasting plasma glucose test. Before brunch in the early hours is the optimal time to provide a blood sample. This test assesses the body's capacity to regulate and sustain glycemic control. When your glucose levels are low, you are immune to the disease.

2. Oral glucose test:

2 hours after your morning meal or noon meal, a lab assistant will draw your blood test. If the results of the test indicate that your glucose level is between 140 and 199 ml/dL, you are pre-diabetic. If the number is less than 140, you are exempt. If your testing results show that you are pre-diabetic, don't worry; there are still methods to stop the disease.

HOW TO REVERSE THE SYMPTOMS OF DIABETES

1. Daily exercise: If you have pre diabetic symptoms, it is crucial that you start exercising every day. This will help your muscles become less dependent on insulin and will help maintain your blood sugar level. Put aside 30 – 45 minutes a day for exercise. To rectify the signs, reduce your intake of simple carbohydrates, which the body will decompose into fat and calories which will be changed into fat. You must consume complex carbohydrates daily, such as millet flour bread, wheat flour, brown pasta, brown rice, and mashed potatoes. White bread, confectionery, chocolate, pasta, rice, cookies, and cake should be avoided.

2. Consumes copious amounts of water: Hydrate and consume 8 to 10 containers of water per day to flush toxins from the body via urination.

3. Change to a raising diet: Fiber also lowers your glucose levels but also aids in weight reduction. A diet high in fiber and liquids will allow you to feel satisfied without increasing your blood sugar. Legumes, fresh fruits and vegetables contain an abundance of fiber.

4. Avoid high stress levels: If you want to rectify your diabetes symptoms, users should prevent excessive stress. Practice yoga, experiment with meditation, and get ample rest. These are the natural, side-effect-free methods to combat early diabetes. To avoid diabetes, adhere to a balanced diet, engage in daily exercise, and check what you consume.

DIABETES AND THE HUMAN METHOD

The pancreas contains three distinct cell types: alpha-cells, beta-cells, and delta-cells. These generate various enzymes for managing blood sugar levels.

- The cells congregate together apex predator generate carbohydrate hormone, which raises blood sugar levels
- Beta-cells cause diabetes, which reduces glucose uptake;

- Delta-cells generate somatostatin, which regulates Alpha and Beta cells. Diabetes is characterized by impaired beta-cell function and constant elevated blood sugar levels.

DIABETES MANAGEMENT AND CURE

Several botanicals have been discovered to be highly successful in treating diabetes and reducing blood sugar levels. The most significant benefit of these natural diabetes medications is their ability to reduce blood sugar levels. The primary benefit of such herbal diabetes remedies is their lack of no negative side effects. Below is a list of many of the greatest effective botanicals for treating diabetes.

1. Bitter gourd: is considered the most effective treatment for diabetes. Daily consumption of at least one spoonful of bitter gourd liquid reduces blood and urine glucose levels. Having bitter gourd prepared with delight for a duration of three months will significantly reduce diabetes.

2. A combination of one tablespoon of Indian gooseberry juice and one cup of fresh bitter gourd juice, consumed daily for two months, will stimulate insulin production by the pancreas.

3. Fresh water containing 10 tulsi leaves: Consuming 10 mint plants and 10 belptras on an empty stomach first thing in the morning helps control blood sugar levels. Mix and pulverize fenugreek seeds (100 grams), turmeric (50 grams), and white peppers. Consume one spoonful of this powder twice daily with such a milky beverage. Place one teaspoon of water into a metal container at night and consume the water the following morning.

NUTRITIONAL PREPARATION FOR DIABETES

Diabetes is a disease that can be significantly exacerbated by a poor diet. Consequently, diet preparation is the centerpiece of diabetes management. Avoid sugar in any form; rice, potato, banana, cereals, and fruits with a high sugar content should be avoided. Each meal should include at least one astringent dish. Green veggies, black wheat, soy, fish, etc., should be consumed in abundance. Bitter gourd, beans, cucumber, onion, and garlic, Indian blackberry, Jambul fruit, grapes, and cereals such as Bengal wheat and black wheat ought to be part of the diet. Raw vegetables and botanicals contribute to pancreatic stimulation and increased insulin production.

CHAPTER FOUR

NATURAL MEANS TO DIABETES CONTROL

1. CURRY LEAVES FOR HYPERGLYCEMIA

It's considerably safer to use a natural approach for managing diabetes. Curry leaves regulate oxidative stress and carbohydrate metabolism. Additionally, curry leaves stimulate insulin production by modulating glucose levels in the blood. If you have diabetes, simply consume 8 to 10 fresh curry leaves each morning for approximately three months. Consuming 10 curry leaves in the morning promotes healthy weight loss in obese diabetics and also reduces fat levels.

2. CUCUMBER FRUIT

Cucumber helps diabetics reduce their blood glucose levels. Foods that contain an abundance. Carbohydrates can induce unwelcome blood sugar spikes. In contrast, high-fiber, low-sugar, and low-carbohydrate diets can help reduce blood sugar levels. As a non-starchy, high water-content, and fiber-rich vegetable. Cucumbers may assist in blood sugar regulation, it's also contains only 0.9 grain of carbohydrate and 1.7 grain of sugar per cup serving. As stated by the American Diabetes Association, non-starchy foods such as cucumbers are

unlikely to raise blood sugar levels.
Moreover, one drink of cucumbers
has just 16 energies and 0.5 grams of
soluble fiber. Cucumbers can allow
you to boost your fiber intake without
significantly increasing your calorie
intake.

3. FLUID CONTENT

When blood levels of glucose are
excessive, water is essential for
removing excess sugar from the body.
Since more than 95% of a cucumber's
weight is water.

4. INSULIN PLANT

Its scientific name is Chamaecostus
cuspidatus, and its common name is
the burning costus or spiral flag. As
implied by their name, insulin leaves

are indispensable as an herbal
treatment for diabetics.

- Anti-Bacteria
- e-coli microbes (digestive tract) increasing defense, decreasing hypertension
- scratchy throat treatment
- urinary tract health
- kidney septicity
- kidney pebble
- liver disorder

How to prepare insulin leaves for infusion/tea

The best method to prepare diabetes foliage is by simmering the leaves in water; pay close attention to the subsequent instructions and explanation to learn how to make a medicinal herbs drink from insulin leaves that can be done at home.

- Handpicked ten or more glucagon leaves
- Slice the foliage
- Dehydrate the foliage
- The leaf extract is now prepared to be steeped in a teapot
- Boil the water until it is boiling and put the insulin leaves into the glass
- Carry the boiling water and then add each teaspoon of glucagon foliage to the tumbler.

Wait till the liquid in the glass changes color to brown.

- Add pure honey for a more delicate and fragrant flavor. Every day, consume a sufficient amount of liquids.

5. MIRACLE SEED

This seed, known as ABERE in the Yoruba language of Nigeria, is so potent that it treats countless maladies for which we would otherwise spend a great deal of money. Such a seed's type species is Hunteria unbellata. This kernel is utilized to treat diabetes in herbal medicine.

Preparation

- Slice forty seeds and marinate them in coconut water overnight.
- Take two teaspoons of the mixture three times daily
- A further technique includes cloves
- Abere seed (hunteria umbellata) and one liter of coconut water
- Grind clove and hunteria umbellata together (the same quantity)
- Put one spoonful of the solution and a liter of coconut water

Dosage

A daily dose

6. LICORICE IN THE FIGHT AGAINST DIABETES

Although medicinal treatments are frequently used to cure diseases, individuals do not avoid the disease from developing and have numerous adverse effects. However, licorice root is an efficient and organic alternative to the same drugs that can inhibit the progression of the disease, manage its effects, and then almost entirely eradicate its signs.

Effect of licorice root on glucose levels:

Researchers administered a 60-day dose of licorice root to diabetic rats and observed a reduction in their blood glucose levels. The results demonstrated that licorice phenolic content decreased glucose levels, recovered kidney function, and slowed losing weight. In addition, the supplement restored the Kidney's antioxidant potential, efficiently erasing all diabetics' detrimental effects on their systems and promoting recovery. Due to its inflammatory and glucose concentrations characteristics, licorice root extract has the potential to have a similar effect on diabetics and produce a major decrease in blood glucose concentrations.

What effect the natural components in licorice root have on diabetic patients

It was discovered that the licorice root contains an active substance known as amorfrutin, which not only regulates and reduces blood sugar levels, but is also mildly effective as an anti-inflammatory, and is therefore helpful in avoiding fatty liver disease, which is a very common condition caused by, among other things, malnutrition. The amorfrutin compounds adhere to receptors in the cell's central nervous system and have an advantageous impact on the amount of lipids and glucose, thereby lowering the level and preventing the danger of developing insulin sensitivity inside the body, one of the primary causes of the development of diabetes. A therosderosis, for which licorice root may be an effective natural treatment. The medicinal properties and qualities of licorice root aid diabetics. It has been established that no more than 0.2 grams of licorice root extract per day for 12 months can result in a substantial decrease in total cholesterol LDL and blood pressure, so that licorice has an important addition to the decrease of Cholesterol and other learned disorders.

7. YOGHURT FOR DIABETES

Yogurt and its effect on glucose levels, in addition to some studies concerning type 2 diabetes. According to studies, yogurt consumption is linked with a 17% lower incidence of type 2 diabetes. It is essential to observe, however, that the yogurt should not be sugar-sweetened or arterially a yogurt that has been seasoned. For the most advantages of a good plain, full-fat yogurt contains relatively low levels of natural sugars, as well as moderate fat and essential fats, which serve to regulate blood sugar, appetite, and hormone balance. Furthermore, the advantageous microbes in a high-quality plain, full-fat yoghurt help to promote digestive health, which is of great benefit to diabetics. If you prefer foods that are a little sweeter, add very little sugar or monk fruit sweetener to your basic filled yogurt, along with a handful of fresh or dried strawberries along with a few pumplain seeds or nuts for a delectable and well-balanced lunch or snack that controls blood sugar and promotes fat loss. Regarding blood glucose diabetes, if you believe that this form of diabetes is irreversible, as many misguided physicians will advise you, then you must provide evidence on how to effectively cure type 2 - diabetes.

Ingredients

- Packet of cardamom
- Pure garlic
- Fresh ginger

- Honey

Preparation

Cardamom stick ground to yield one teaspoon extract, garlic and ginger ground to yield one teaspoon

Combine half a teaspoon of each mixture in a cup, add one teaspoon of honey and 1/2 cup of tepid water, and consume twice daily.

8. STEVIA PLANT

After digestion, all sugars and carbohydrates are converted to glucose, which is then circulated throughout the body for absorption by tissues and organs to fuel their activity. Diabetes lacks the necessary process for this glucose uptake, and as a result, the remaining sugar is depleted. It is more serious if blood glucose does not remain inactive, as it then begins to attack the enzymes that make up the body systems and organs, resulting in their dysfunction. This explains why diabetics typically mature faster and are susceptible to a variety of health problems. What if we could avoid excessive blood sugar and discover alternative ways to power the cells? The plant contains steviol glycoside, which really is approximately one hundred times sweeter than table sugar. Now that the body cannot utilize the glycoside in stevia, it contains zero calories and is an ideal sugar substitute for diabetics. It's fascinating that it was found that this species has been common among Asians, particularly the Japanese, who are known for their broad acceptance of natural supplements for decades. Several nations have authorized the consumption of stevia as a food additive, while others are still conducting tests. In regions in which the shrub is plentiful, it is known as sweet herb and is used as a common sweetener in teas and cuisines. In Japan, stevia is widely used for domestic, industrial, and business reasons, with a variety of businesses producing and refining the essence of the plants for domestic use, as most foods begin to phase out artificial sweeteners due to claims of their high toxicity.

9. MANGO FOLIAGE FOR DIABETES

Diabetes can be effectively managed with mango leaves. Take mango leaves, soak them in water and keep it overnight. Early morning on a vacant stomach, consume the solution. You can also take it in powder form.

Dry the leaves of mango and make it into powder, mix the dried powder, one teaspoon of mango leaves in a glass of water and drink on empty stomach every morning. You can as well boil the mango leaves to prepare herbal tea. Take the herbal tea, one cup on empty stomach in the morning and one cup at night.

10. SOURSOP AGAINST DIABETES

Soursop assists in maintaining and regulating a stable glucose level. This inhibits a decrease in glucose levels in the blood. Here, acerogenin performs an important role. A study published in the journal of traditional medicine and dietary supplements has provided scientific evidence for this advantage. According to the study, consuming soursop can help treat diabetes. In cases of diabetes or Spasin, it can also be consumed as an infusion of soursop roots and foliage.

Preparation

Heat 40 to 50 soursop leaves and approximately 2 liters of water. Once prepared, allow the solution to settle for just a minute, then consume three portions per day. Perform it frequently for the best results.

11. FIG LEAVES TO CURE DIABETES AND LUNG INFLAMMATION

Figs are abundant in a wide range of beneficial polyphenolic nutrients and antioxidants, whether they are fresh or dried. The initial fruits our ancient ancestors relished was the sweet fig. The grown fig seems to have the appearance of a ring or a pear, and its flesh is succulent.

Health benefits

1. Figs contain soluble food fibers, minerals and vitamins.

2. Fresh figs are valued for their abundance of antioxidants such as carotene, vitamin, lutein and chromogenic acid.

3. Fresh figs contain high levels of antioxidants protects us from free radicals whose destructive activity can lead to premature aging, dementia, heart disease and cancer.

4. Figs, as well as other fiber rich foods, helps to lose weight and maintain the desired weight.

5. Anti-carcinogenic compounds include benzaldehyde and counmarins are found in figs. Preliminary medical

research has confirmed the potential action of these compounds on prostate and skin carcinoma.

6. Fig solve the problems of curly eyes and nipple pains. Overnight place a half-sliced fresh fig in the painful area and remove the fig in the morning and wash your feet with hot water.

7. Dried figs are a highly concentrated source of mineral, vitamins, and antioxidants. They have more calories than fresh. 249 calories per hundred grams. Both fresh and dry figs contain a significant amount of B vitamins such as niacin, pyridoxine, pantothenic and folic acid. The breakdown of amino acids,

carbohydrates, and lipids. The B complex is significant for the brain function, especially for good mood.

8. Dried figs are an abundant source of minerals of calcium, zinc, potassium, selenium, iron, and copper-iron and copper are needs to create red blood cells, white potassium is an important component of cells and body fluids, and helps regulate heart rhythm and blood pressure.

9. Cooking figs like tea helps with brain disease, inflammation of the throat and lungs.

10. The leaves from figs are medical and has long been known for their medicinal properties. It treats

bronchitis, nipples problems, liver cirrhosis, high blood pressure, skin problems and sores.

But the novelty is that fig leaves are also extremely good for diabetes. Use fig leaf juice immediately with breakfast. You can also boil the fig leaves in the water and drink as tea.

How to prepare tea from fig leaf

Pour two teaspoon of dried fig leaves with a cup (200ml) of boiling water. Cover and leaves for 10 – 15 minutes. Every morning, have a glass of this tea at breakfast.

HERBS FOR DIABETICS

- Green tea

- Dandelion

- Cactus

- Moringa

- Garlic tea

- Black seeds

- Cinnamon tea

- Turmeric tea

- Ginger

- Bitter cola

- Garlic

- Clove

preparation

Mix a ½ tea spoon of each of the

herbs and drink an hour after lunch.

For Garlic tea, Black seeds,

Cinnamon tea and Turmeric tea mix

½ tea spoon of each of the herbs and

drink before sleeping.

Other diabetes herbs:

- Bitter leaves
- Scent leaves
- Neem leaves
- 3 bulb of onion
- Garlic
- Little potash

Preparation

Squeeze the leaves of bitter leaves, scent leaves and neem leaves.

Blend the onion, garlic, and mix with the juice obtained from the leaves add grinded little potash to it.

Dosage

Adult 3 spoon thrice daily and children 1 spoon thrice daily

HERBAL DETOXIFICATION FOR DIABETES PATIENT

If you are suffering from diabetes and have been on medication for long, you probably want to detoxify to save your kidneys, get yourself chlorophyll juice. After every meal mix Okra beverages

- Cactus tea
- Saw palmetto
- Dandelion
- Cup of hot water
- Black seed
- Green tea
- Okra beverage tea
- Fenugreek tea
- Guaiac tea

Preparation

To make the herbal tea, get a ½ teaspoon of each of the herbs and put 750mls of hot water and allow the herbs to cool

Dosage

Take 250ml of the herbal drink 3 times a day. 30 minutes after meal. For results, have a bowl of vegetables and proteins as your meals and reduce starchy food until your body is good enough to metabolize and utilize glucose in your body.

Other diabetes cure:

1. This remedy for diabetes will also make your system clean and clear without sickness. Get the root of lime tree and cut it into pieces, put it in an

empty keg of 2 litters, add 7 or 9 negro pepper, add water day. Take 2 or 3 times daily.

2. Squeeze bitter leave, scent leave and pawpaw leaves together. Add some grinded garlic. Drink twice daily for 3 weeks One glass cup or half before meal in the morning and after meal in the evening.

3. Boil all the recipes above Guava leaves, Mango leaves, Mango seed and Avocado leaves
 in 3 litters of water. Take three time daily.

4. Soak spring onion leaves and okra in water overnight. Drink first on empty stomach in the following morning.

5. INGREDIENTS

- Wheat 100gm

- Barley 100gm

- Black seed 100gm

Method of preparation

- Put all the above ingredients in 5 cups of water.

- Boil it for 10 minutes

- Allow it to cool down when it has cold,

- Filter out the seeds and preserve the solution in a glass jug or bottle.

Dosage

Take one small cup of this solution every day early in the morning on an empty stomach for seven days. Repeat the same in the following week but on alternate days. Within these 2 weeks of treatment, you will wonder to see that you have been cured diabetes life style.

- Avoid sleeping during day time
- Avoid smoking
- Take adequate eye care
- Do exercise regularly
- Take extra care of your foot

CHAPTER FIVE

STUMPY BLOOD PRESSURE HYPOGLYCEMIA

Hypoglycemia is a condition in which the circulatory system sugar level is below the normal range. It usually means blood sugar less than 70mg/dh.

CAUSES

- Taking too much insulin
- Skipping a meal
- Exercising too strenuously
- Drinking too much alcohol (in people with diabetes)
- Critical or organ failure (kidney, heart or liver)
- Hormone deficiencies
- Tumors.

- Fasting

- Inherited abnormalities

- Lack of appropriate diet

- Recovery from gastrointestinal surgery

- Prolonged illness

- Autoimmune disorder

- Certain medication such as quinolonec, pentamidine, quinine, beta-blocker, angiotensin- converting anzyme agents and IGF.

SYMPTOMS

Among the signs of insufficient blood sugar are:

- Fatigue

- Increase appetite

- Cloudy thinking

- Blurry vision

- Headache

- Excessive sweating

- Dizziness

- Trembling, lack of
  concentration

- Depression, anxiety

- Mental confusion, irritability

- Heart palpitation

- Slurred speech

- Seizures

- Fatigue

- Pale facial complexion

It is essential to test your sugar levels
as soon as you experience these

symptoms to determine if you are

suffering from diabetes.

You might get these signs whenever

your blood sugar drops rapidly. Once

it has been determined that the blood

sugar level has decreased compared to

regular, you must consume basic

glucose with minimal or no fiber. You

ought to avoid foods that are high in

fat. The fat that typically stabilizes

blood sugar levels after a meal can

actually slow the body's absorption of

these essential simple carbohydrates.

Glucose pills or glucose gel are the

most commonly prescribed therapy

for low blood sugar. However, raising

your blood sugar quickly is the

primary goal. But what could

adequately treat low blood sugar is what should be our concern rather than to result to chalky tablets filled with processed sugar food coloring and artificial flavor. The following are natural ways of treating hypoglycemia:

1. All natural peanut: Peanut butter or any nut butter without added sugar is filled with protein and fat and can help alleviate these symptoms without raising your blood sugar. This remedy is good for someone whose blood sugar is greater than 80mg/dl but feeling symptoms of hypoglycemia.

2. Peanut spread and crackers: When the blood level is between 70 and 80

mg/dL, your bloodstream sugar is strictly not insufficient. In this instance, the cracker will help elevate the glucose levels in your blood gradually, while the peanut butter's fat and protein will maintain them.

3. If the glucose level in your blood is between 55 and 70 mg/dl, you require a few things:

- Raisin
- Medjooldates
- Cupplesauce
- Bananas
- Grapes
- Pineapple

All of the items outlined above are either freshly picked or dried fruits that contain more organically produced glucose than other fruits. While these do contain some fiber, the amount is negligible, and they will rapidly and effectively elevate blood sugar levels.

4. If your blood sugar is less than 55mg/dl you will need the following:

- Grape pulp
- Honey and syrup made from maple.

Fiber, lipids, and protein should not be present. Grape juice is one of the most carbohydrate-rich beverages and is highly beneficial for patients with hypoglycemia who have reached the age of seventy. Some individuals have difficulty chewing and ingesting if their glucose levels exceeds this point, so we should concentrate on condensed forms of glucose such as high-carbohydrate juices or sweeteners such as natural maple syrup and honey to taste.

NUTRITION AND SUPPLEMENTS FOR HYPOGLYCEMIA.

Food to avoid

1. Eliminate suspected food allergens such as diary milk, cheese, and ice cream, wheat (gluten), soy, corn, preservatives and chemical food additives.

2. Avoid refined foods such as white bread, pastas and sugar unless you

need them for an immediate blood sugar increase.

3. Eliminate trans fatty acids found in commercially baked goods such as cookies, cakes, French fries, onion rings, donuts, processed foods and margarine.

4. Avoid alcohol and tobacco, lower caffeine intake, as caffeine impacts several conditions and medications.

DIETS FOR HYPOGLYCEMIA

1. Eat food high in B- vitamins and iron such as whole grains, fresh vegetables and sea vegetables.

2. Consume antioxidant-rich foods, such as cranberries, cherries, and tomatoes, as well as zucchini and green peppers.

3. Soluble fiber such as flaxseed and pure oat bran can slow the rate at which dietary sugars enter the blood and help regulate blood sugars throughout the day. Consume 1 to 3 tablespoon of either of these fiber sources before meals with a full glass of water.

4. Utilize healthful fats for cooking like virgin olive oil and oil from coconuts

HERBAL REMEDIES

1. GREEN BREW (camellia sinensis)

For antioxidants effect, you can prepare teas from the leaf of this herb.

2. PURE PARSLEY (ocimum sanctum)

For stress balance, you can prepare teas from the plant. Holy basil slow blood clothing and therefore increase the effect of blood-thinning medicines.

3. ACUPUNCTURE

Acupuncture may decrease stress, increase coping skills and regulate hormone function.

4. LICORICE ROOT

Boil few pieces of licorice in water for 5-10 minutes' strain and allow it to cool. Drink a cup of this mixture once a day.

5. DANDELION ROOTS

Dandelion roots are rich in calcium that helps in proper functioning of liver and pancreas. This alternative therapy for low levels of sugar assists in regulating the amount of sugar in the blood to avoid diabetes.

How to prepare

Powder the dandelion roots and stir it add two spoons of the powder in a glass of warm milk. Drink this daily for better results.

Alternatively, a concoction of the roots can also be made and consumed regularly.

6. TOMATOES

Extract the juice from 4 -5 tomatoes drink 2 glasses of tomatoes juice every day. Add fresh tomatoes to diet.

7. SUNFLOWER SEEDS

Include raw sunflower seeds in salads. Powdered sunflower seeds can be taken along with water.

8. BARLEY

Barley is an excellent food for people suffering from type 2 diabetes. It is rich in minerals vitamins and dietary fibers which maintains the glucose level in the blood. It contains magnesium and beta-glucan which helps in regulating the glucose absorption in the blood.

Preparation

Prepare oatmeal from barley cereals. Two to three times per day, based on the degree of low blood sugar, consume barley liquid.

HOW FOODS ARE ABLE TO INCREASE BLOOD PRESSURE QUICK

A plantation of produce such as banana, apple, or orange

- 2 teaspoons of yeast extract

- 15 plums

- Half a cup of an apple, orange, pineapple or berry juice from a fruit

- Half cup ordinary beverage (not sugary free)

- One cup fat Reduced milk

- One teaspoon of sugar or jam

- 15 Biscuits

FOODS WITH HIGHER SUGAR

- Watermelon

- Dried dates

- Pineapple

- Ripe banana

- Fruit juice: the center of disease controls and prevention (CDC) stated that drinking fruit juice during a meal or on its own quickly raises a person's blood sugar level.

AFRICAN HERBS FOR HYPOGLYCEMIA

The following flora have anti-diabetic properties:

- Eriocephalus punctulatus

- The species Hyposis hemerocallides

- African Spud

- Dicoma anomale

- Morella serreta

- Gazania krebsiana

- Elephatorrliza elephantina

- Hermanniac pinnate inborn

- Commeline Afro-American

- Haplocerpha scapose

- Helicysum aureum

- Empodium plicatum

- Minulus gracilis

- Pentamisia pruneloides

- Cannabis sativa

- Bulbine narcissifolic

- Rumex lanceoletus

- Gunnera perpense
- Aloe vera
- Asparagus asparagoides
- The species Anthosperium jernatu
- Erythine zeyheri
- The species Sisymbrium theellingi
- Momordica charantis
- Chinese Coptis

EFFICACY OF HYPOGLYCEMIA HERBS

The efficacy of hypoglycemia herbs that has been mediated by increasing insulins secretion (ginseng, bitter melons, aloes, brophytum, sentitinum). Boosting fatty and muscle insulin absorption.

DAILY THERAPIES FOR HYPOGLYCEMIA

1. Take saltier foods and drink a lot of water

2. Chew alligator pepper and bitter cola

3. Putting raw Nopal cactus with orange juice and pineapple juice in a fruit smoothie every morning.

4. Beetroot works wonder just blend the beetroot with the stem and leaf and drink. You can add honey to it

5. Honey, sugar cane juice and fruit juice are good for you

6. Incorporate garden egg leaves and the seeds into your diet.

7. Blend two handful of fresh leaves of sweet potato is one liter of water and drink two glasses daily for five days.

8. Boil the bark stem of mahogany plant in water with sugar. Drink morning and night.

9. Always take dates, bananas and sugar cane

10. You can be taking soft drink such as sprite, coke or Pepsi as well

11. Take oral glucose